# The Fasting path

By

MELVIS MICHAEL

# Table of contents

Title page.................................1

Copyright page.........................2

Table of contents......................3

Let's go....................................4

Outline......................................5

**Chapter 1**

The science of fasting.............6

**Chapter 2**

The mental side of fasting......8

**Chapter 3**

Defeating Hunger......................9

**Chapter 4**

Calories Restriction and Food Types.........................................10

**Chapter 5**

Contemplating food..................12

**Chapter 6**

Planning to fast.........................14

**Chapter 7**

Straightforward fasting............17

**Chapter 8**

Skipping Meals.......................... 18

**Chapter 9**

Work out ...................................20

**Chapter 10**

Monitoring Progress..................22

**Chapter 11**

Incidental Effects.........................23

**Chapter 12**

Incorporating Fasting Into Your Way of Life
...............................................25

About the Author ..................... 28

# Let's go

# Outline

Irregular fasting is turning out to be more and more famous. Life in the Fasting path (2022) is a jump into each part of fasting for weight control and by and large wellbeing. Melvis Michael offers her involvement in fasting, she also makes sense of the science and exposes the legends, and tolls in with hints that her patients have pragmatically adhered to and they've worked for them. Presently, she's educating perusers about the advantages, feasts, and schedules of irregular fasting.

# The Science of Fasting

My friend was threatened by science, which is the reason she was fat for almost all her life. She battled with a huge number of medical issues, including fruitlessness and sinus contaminations. She followed physicians' instructions and, surprisingly, shed pounds, however it continuously returned, until she had a go at fasting. Eating less frequently implied that her body had an additional opportunity to consume energy. Her medical problems are presently gone, and she has at long last made due to reach and keep up with her objective weight. While weight doesn't characterize whether you are metabolically solid or not, fasting altogether diminishes metabolic conditions like, sort 2 diabetes. The body has two different ways of putting away food. To begin with, sugar is accessible for fast energy use. The second, muscle-to-fat ratio, is possibly utilized when the body doesn't have glucose left. Insulin is the chemical that tells the body when it necessities to change over food into energy. Consuming carbs, for instance, will spike blood sugar levels. Subsequently, insulin levels will likewise spike. These significant levels are what keep fat from being singed. In the long run, insulin is not generally as expected created, and that is the point at which you foster sort 2 diabetes. In general, fasting assumes a gigantic part in directing chemicals. At the point when you are fasting, low insulin levels signal that the body needs to consume fat. Accordingly, fasting is the most sensible approach to losing and keeping up weight.

# The Mental Side of Fasting

The resultant effects from fasting is not just physical. At the point when you shed pounds and discard all the unbearable symptoms of overflow fat, you normally become more euphoric. Exactly when you at first beginning fasting, you could experience some irritability due to changes in synthetic substances and fluctuating proportions of electrolytes while losing water weight. These, regardless, are available second influences.

Excess weight makes a lot of upsetting isolation. Overweight people are often considered to be dormant, but that stems from a lie. Another piece of deception is that fundamentally eating less and moving more is a strong framework. It's the most typical dietary direction, and it's misguided. Fasting, regardless, is a possible lifestyle. It is unobtrusive and basic, as you don't need to contribute to presumably better food things. It's furthermore staggeringly versatile, and you can alter your plan according to your regular presence.

## Defeating Hunger

However hunger frequently appears to be a major domineering jerk,
it is only a propensity. When you start eating less, hunger will menace you less habitually. You'll notice that when you're eager, however, don't eat, the craving, at last, dies down. You can mollify hunger by basically drinking water.
Appetite ought not to be mistaken for starvation. Your body has a lot of provisions to use. Hunger is constrained by satiety chemicals and stretch receptors in the stomach. At the point when food extends the stomach enough, satiety chemicals are delivered, and keeping on eating after that is difficult. We in reality get eager at specific times on the grounds that we are accustomed to eating at those times. The wave of appetite will ultimately pass, in light of the fact that the body can deal with itself by consuming the fat it has put away. To get out from under your yearning propensities,just eat at the table, and begin drinking water rather than eating your typical nibble at a particular time.

## Calorie Restriction and Food Types

Calorie impediment is totally misleading we truly need to fight.

The "Calories In, Calories Out" approach to weight decrease has a victory speed of around 1 percent. A container of pop and an unobtrusive pack of rough almonds have a comparable number of calories. Regardless, our bodies cycle them very surprisingly. Soda will spike your glucose levels, but almonds will not. That is the explanation calories have no effect.

Another ordinary legend is the gamble of evading a dining experience. Before the 1980s, the norm was three meals regular, and it was fine to skip one expecting that you felt like it. The primary thing that will happen to expect you to skirt a dining experience is that your body will consume the fat it has taken care of. This misrepresentation is a consequence of commercialization. Fasting was morerecognized previously, and numerous people avoided it for severe reasons. Snacking was glared upon. Today, the rotundity crisis is roaring, yet snacking is enabled.

Instead of standard reasoning, fasting has a ton to do with the type of food you're consuming.

While specific people can speedy actually furthermore, keep a strong burden while still eating a lot of treats, this isn't valid for everyone. Intermittent fasting and a strong diet merged are fantastic. To stay in fasting path, a low-carb diet stacked with strong fats is the best approach. Carbs cause a sugar spike in the blood, which is what we want to avoid. You shouldn't focus on counting carbs, yet endeavor to avoid food sources like treats, white bread, pasta, rice, potatoes, beans, and natural items. In light of everything, eat more vegetables, nuts, berries, meats, and dairy.

## Contemplating Food

Hankering your number one pastry can drive you insane. You really want to begin pondering food in an unexpected way. Cut off any close-to-home associations you have with food, and consider it a simple wellspring of energy. You shouldn't see food as a prize, as a solace, or as a companion to run to when circumstances become difficult. To change your attitude, begin recording how you felt while eating every food consistently, and why you consumed it.

Now and again delight transforms into a habit, what's more, it is extremely simple to get dependent on handled food varieties, as sugar produces dopamine in the cerebrum very much like heroin does. You needn't bother with food to interface with friends and family, and you needn't bother with desserts to assuage pressure. Dependence is essential for daily practice, and you can embrace elective schedules that incorporate taking a shower, work out, head out to the motion pictures, going on a walk, and contemplating.

## Planning to Fast

The start of your fasting journey may be energizing however harrowing. Assuming you've had food issues previously, you might question your capacity too quickly. Fasting is more straightforward than you

think.
Fantasies about fasting are excessively normal.
Fasting won't make you debilitated. It, as a matter of fact, brings down your possibility of creating quite a large number of infections. Fasting doesn't cause your blood sugar levels to crash, it controls them. It doesn't dial back your digestion, and
you will not starve to death. You need to zero in on your objectives and acknowledge them
at the point when they change. Youmight need to contend in a marathon, cut down on meds, or
just concentrate all the more without any problem. Continuously keep your objectives before you.
When you understand what your objectives are and step-by-step instructions to accomplish them, think about cleaning your home. This implies getting rid of any enticing food varieties. Begin putting away veggies on lovely plates, furthermore, you will be more eager to eat them.
Having an emotionally supportive network is vital.
Tell your loved ones what you're doing. They ought to have the option to spur you, also, it could try and lead them to nibble less. If you are fasting with an accomplice, remember that male and female bodies respond in an unexpected way to fasting. Men as a rule lose more weight at

first. However, in the long run, the ladies get up to speed, and the two of them begin losing a portion of a pound of fat for every fasting day.

Research on how fasting and sex associate is nearly non-existent, however, ladies have revealed expanded sex drive after a couple of long periods of fasting. Fasting additionally may help at the point when a lady is attempting to get pregnant, and it might forestall difficulties that could result from the expanded weight. Notwithstanding, fasting is not suggested during pregnancy.

## Straightforward Fasting

Assuming command of when you eat and when is one of the simplest spots to begin your weight reduction venture. You can begin gradually with what is called basic or languid fasting. Change your fasting plan consistently, yet remain predictable. Begin simply by skirting your standard thing snacks. After you become acclimated to that, you can begin cutting feasts. At the point when you begin fasting, having drinks other than water like espresso or on the other hand tea is suggested. You want to keep up with sound sodium levels to remain hydrated.

Some other fasting preparing wheels incorporate vegetable stock, lemon water, and pickle juice. To quit eating, ensure the three feasts you're eating get you full. You might be eating eight times each day, which is a troublesome propensity to break. During your most memorable week, begin eating multiple times all things considered, and go from there. You can decide to eat less, however, you can't decide to be less eager. Eating doesn't forestall appetite and it's experimentally not important to nibble as our bodies don't require it.

## Skipping Meals

After you've effectively kicked eating, the subsequent stage is to skip breakfast. Around evening time, make sure your supper is loaded with food sources that will fill you up, and keep away from ones that will make you feel hungrier toward the beginning of the day, likesugars.

The following day, you will be ravenous, yet entirely as it were since your body anticipates breakfast. You will before long become acclimated to not eating. Later you do, you are prepared to begin skipping lunch.

While having just supper begins feeling simple, begin eating just two days of the week.

You can pick which feasts to skip.

Fasting is profoundly adaptable, and soon you will be prepared for the 36-hour quick. Some individuals find it hard to nod off after a full day of fasting, so ensure you are well hydrated and keep away from screens before bed. The sooner you nod off, the quicker your next feast will come. At the point when you ultimately start fasting for several days, you want to bit by bit break your quick. Eat gradually and carefully for diets longer than five days, and have a nibble before your most memorable large dinner.

# Work out

You want to practice not really for weight reduction, but rather for wellbeing, so working out while fasting is energized. Any kind of action is great, whether you're strolling the canine or going up the multiple times. Anything that will get your heart rolling is viewed as exercise. Plan your activity as per your timetable also, capacities. Ensure that whatever you're doing is agreeable, and think about strength preparing. When you become accustomed to a certain schedule, zest it up. That implies you're getting more grounded.

Devouring

Fasting eventually makes eating more agreeable. After each quick, you can eat. Nonetheless, that doesn't mean eating garbage food until you can move no more. Devouring implies eating charming good food over a longer timeframe, generally 60 minutes. You need to pick food varieties that you appreciate, that make you feel full, however, that won't cause you to feel slow. A goliath bowl of greens with bacon what's more, cheddar close by a major piece of sizzling meat sounds awesome. You ought to hold back nothing assortment of varieties and surfaces in your dining experience.

Make an occasion out of it, and partake in each nibble. You do not just have the right to eat; you likewise merit to appreciate what you're eating. Eliminate any interruptions like tech and books, and eat until you are easily full.

Be aware of what you're eating, and effectively keep away from food sources that you know you tend to long for. Keep away from the liquor and soft drinks. Get going with the protein and fat on your plate. When you come to the carbs, which are normally individuals' top choices, you will not have a voracious long for them. You ought to likewise never go food shopping when you're eager. You will make more careful choices about what to purchase when you are full.

## Monitoring Progress

During your fasting process, you want to keep tabs on your development and achievement. Really this doesn't simply mean recording how much weight you've lost. Decide a reasonable date for when you'd like to accomplish a specific objective. Write down goal lines where you can really look at your advancement furthermore, celebrate. On the off chance that you don't have a terrible relationship with scales, they can be an extraordinary instrument to follow your weight. What ever is the case, in the situation that you will more often than not fixate on numbers and vacillations, try not to utilize a scale.
Alternate ways of the following achievement incorporate estimating your pulse or your blood sugar, perceiving how long you can hold a board position, and seeing how long it requires for you to run winded.

# Incidental effects

When you begin fasting, your body will experience a lot of changes. Everybody is unique, however, a few normal issues have exceptionally basic causes and arrangements. Terrible breath part of it. It shows that your body consumes fat. It as a rule disappears after a while. Bulging is additionally ordinary, and you can just slice your sodium admission to lessen it. Stoppage can be helped by eating more mixed greens and fiber, and looseness of the bowels by splashing chia seeds in water and drinking it. Unsteadiness, sickness, and exhaustion can be kept away from by remaining hydrated.

To fight fatigue while fasting, there are a lot of things you can do. You can peruse, clean the house, work out, call your companions, diary, go out to shop, or simply hang out in the sun. Nonetheless, there are things you ought to abstain from doing, for example, shopping for food, squandering life via web-based entertainment, cooking, cleaning dishes, going to the shopping center, showing up at gatherings, and getting away. This is on the grounds that they are undeniably associated with food and disorder for sure.

# Incorporating Fasting into Your Way of life

While fasting, you can in any case keep a functioning public activity. Planning is fundamental. Fasting is very adaptable, yet you shouldn't become derailed for a really long time. You really want to take responsibility for when you mess up quickly, also, you ought to make an honest effort to keep up with the balance.

Plan as indicated by your social exercises.

Abstain from fasting when you realize you will be in a setting where food is the headliner, or on the other hand promptly accessible. If you would rather not eat the food served, getting a drink is OK furthermore, simply mingle. You don't owe anybody a clarification on the off chance that they ask you for what reason you're not eating. Simply let them know that you previously ate, what's more, don't carefully describe the situation with individuals you're not near.

You ought to have the option to quick as per your way of life. An illustration of a fair quick is the 24-hour quick three times each week. What's the benefit of this is that you can do it twice back to back, and it is not difficult to consolidate your way of life. Certain individuals like to quick at the same time for 72 hours. On specific events, for example, occasions or excursions, you will not have the option to quick by any stretch of the imagination, and that is totally fine. In any case, you ought to know how to refocus. Irrespective of attempting with so much enthusiasm, sooner or perhaps later, you will stagger. You want to have the option to excuse yourself and gain from your botches. Sort out what compelled you to slip and work on it.

Fasting is a polarizing theme, yet you can continuously find a local area that will uphold you. Hold on until there is a strong motivation behind why you want to educate somebody regarding your fasting.

Ensure you are prepared to answer all their questions. Teach yourself about all viewpoints on fasting. Anticipate pessimistic or close-to-home reactions, yet recollect that this is your decision and your life.

Fasting will allow you to foster associations with things you never truly appreciated.

At the point when an extended get-away, you will begin appreciating

nature and exercises much more than going overboard
on food. You will track down better approaches to celebrate, for example, showing up at shows. You will in any case find
yourself commending with food at times, yet
that is OK since you have worked your
way towards your objectives.

## About the Author

MELVIS MICHAEL is a pharmacist by profession. She's also a writer. She writes on health related topics as well as other fields. One of her books include ," why women can't sleep;women's new mental implosion".

www.ingramcontent.com/pod-product-compliance
Lightning Source LLC
LaVergne TN
LVHW020544160826
845677LV00015B/4193

* 9 7 9 8 8 4 6 1 0 4 0 3 7 *